Better Eyesight
for Busy People

All profits from the sale of this book
will be divided between

Mary's Meals
https://www.marysmeals.org.uk

and Sightsavers
http://www.sightsavers.org/

Better Eyesight for Busy People

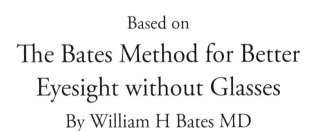

Based on
The Bates Method for Better Eyesight without Glasses
By William H Bates MD

Compiled by
Gillian Snoxall

ISBN: 978-1-78324-039-5

All illustrations by Emily Snape, *www.emilysnape.co.uk*

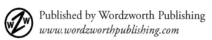
Published by Wordzworth Publishing
www.wordzworthpublishing.com

For Derek,
and for Charles, Paul and Shona
with my love

*"If you do these exercises,
you need never wear glasses again."*

—Mrs I Frewen
Bates Practitioner
Hong Kong 1985

"I no longer bother with glasses."

—Jonathan Barnes
in his excellent book "*Improve Your Eyesight – A Guide
to the Bates Method for Better Eyesight without Glasses*"

Contents

Exercise 1	Getting started	3
Exercise 2	Palming	5
Exercise 3	Sunning	7
Exercise 4	The Big X	9
Exercise 5	Sunnies are a no-no!	11
Exercise 6	Zooming	13
Exercise 7	Blinking	15
Exercise 8	Near and far focusing	17
Exercise 9	Swinging	19
Exercise 10	Circles	21
Exercise 11	Break the staring habit	23
Exercise 12	Outlining	25

Acknowledgements

I remember my surprise when I noticed that our friend Harvey Oates was reading a newspaper in the dim light of the bar in our Club in Hong Kong, without glasses. When I questioned him about this transformation, he explained that he had attended a course of lessons with Mrs I Frewen, a practitioner of the Bates system of natural vision improvement, as a result of which he no longer used glasses at all.

I lost no time in signing up with Mrs Frewen, but unfortunately she was not well at the time and was about to leave Hong Kong. Nevertheless, she did give me a handful of exercises, all of which I have practised almost every day since. Doing these exercises has resulted in my having excellent eyesight and, at the age of 78, I can still read even small print without glasses.

I am profoundly grateful to these three life-changers: the late Dr William Horatio Bates MD (1860–1931) who invented the system; to Mrs I Frewen, Bates Practitioner who started me off on the exercises; and to Harvey Oates for leading me to them.

Introduction

This compilation of easy but effective eye exercises is for all those busy people who would like to improve their eyesight naturally, but who do not have time to wade through acres of print.

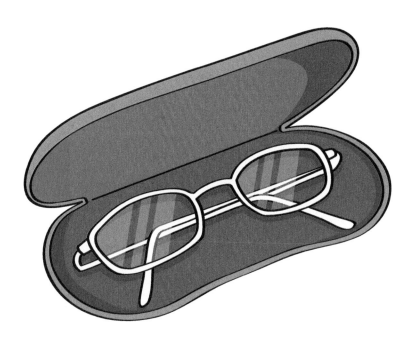

EXERCISE 1

Getting started

**Do without your glasses
as much as you possibly can.**

Resist the urge to put on your glasses first thing in the morning. During the day, remove them whenever you do not actually need them. At the very least, try to go without using glasses for 15 to 20 minutes per day.

These exercises are presented in large print so you can read them without your glasses.

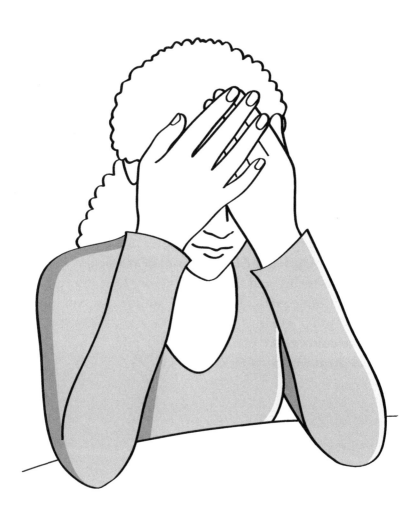

EXERCISE 2

Palming

**Rest your eyes by covering them gently
with your hands, excluding the light,
while relaxing your whole body.**

Try to find a place where you can be peaceful and undisturbed. Close your eyes and cover them gently with your hands, excluding the light while consciously relaxing the whole of your body. Do this for at least five minutes at a time, as often as possible.

Eyesight is closely connected to memory, so while you are palming it is a good idea to picture in your mind's eye a scene which makes you happy. "See" it in detail – the leaves softly rustling in the trees, or the waves washing onto the shore.

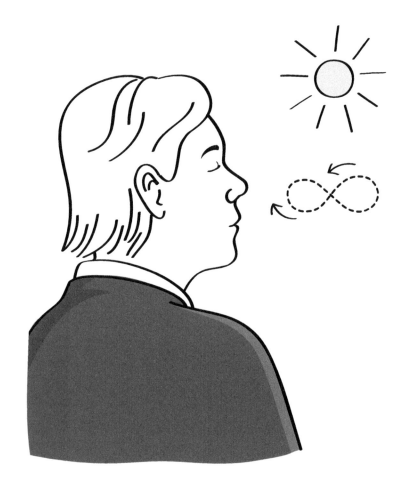

EXERCISE 3

Sunning

With your eyes closed, turn to face the sun and make a horizontal figure-of-eight with your whole head. Then, still with your eyes closed and facing the sun, move your head from side to side, and up and down.

Behind your closed eyelids your eyes will be adjusting to the different angles of the light, and making the small shifts that are so important to strengthening your eye muscles. Start by doing this for half a minute, repeated two or three times.

Over the next week or two, gradually build up the time spent sunning until you are doing it for around five minutes per session, at least once a day if possible. (If there is no sunshine, a strong lamp can be used instead).

Important: Of course, you should *never* look directly at the sun, except with your eyes closed.

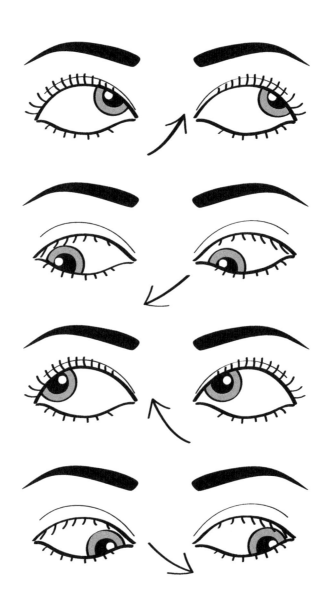

EXERCISE 4

The Big X

Make a big X with your eyes, looking to the top-right as far as you can, then down to the bottom-left as far as possible. Then do the opposite – from top-left to bottom-right. Repeat four times in each direction.

Do this throughout the day, whenever you get the chance.

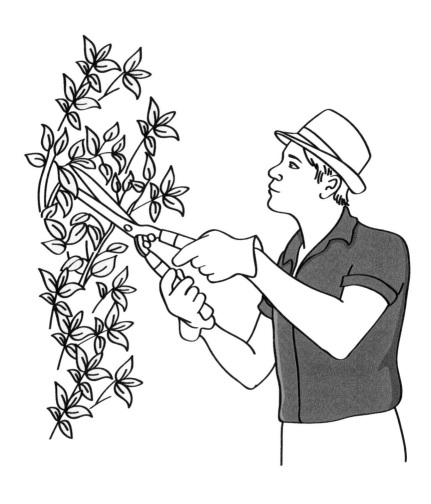

EXERCISE 5

Sunnies are a no-no!

**Do without your sunglasses as
much as you possibly can.**

Your eyes will adjust naturally to the change in light when
you go outdoors, and it is good exercise for them to do so.

The only time you might need sunglasses is when you
are snow-skiing in bright sunshine.

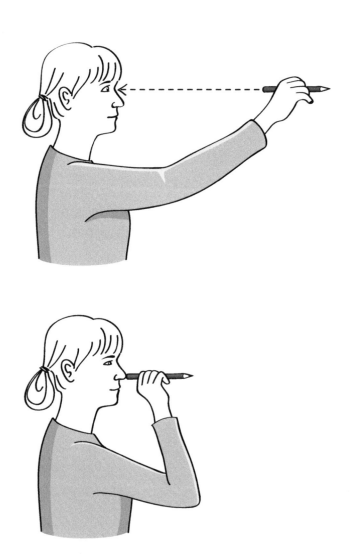

EXERCISE 6

Zooming

Sitting in a comfortable position, hold
a pencil at arm's length in front of you,
with the blunt end towards you.

Focusing on the blunt end all the time, bring
the pencil up to your nose, then take it up
to the top of your forehead, back down over
your nose, mouth and chin to your chest.

Then bring it back up to your nose
and on out to arm's length again.

This exercise will strengthen your eyes' ability to focus, and generally improve your eye muscles. Do it whenever you get the chance.

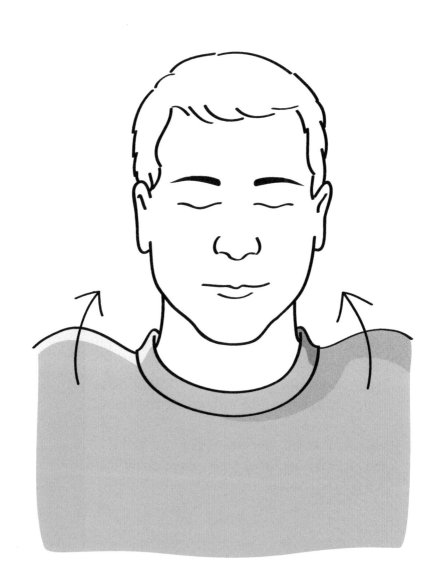

EXERCISE 7

Blinking

**Perform 300 blinks.
Yes, that's right: 300 blinks.**

**At the end of 300 blinks, do a big squeeze
of your eyes, neck and shoulders.**

It is easiest to count the blinks in sets of ten, thus:

One, two, three … ten
One, two, three … twenty
One, two, three … thirty
and so on.

This exercise helps to keep your eyes fresh and better able
to focus. You should do it at least once a day.

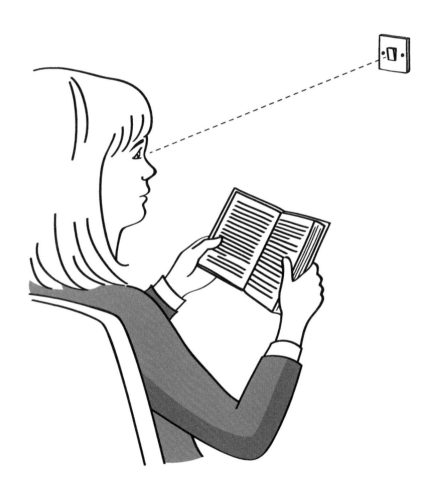

EXERCISE 8

Near and far focusing

**Focus on a nearby object, perhaps
the print of a book you are holding,
then focus on some distant object
such as a light switch on a far wall.**

**Change your focus to the far object and
back to the close one, several times.**

Again, this very beneficial exercise can be done throughout the day, whenever you get the chance. I often do it
while waiting for the traffic lights to change, focusing
on the number-plate of the car in front, then back to a
detail on my steering wheel.

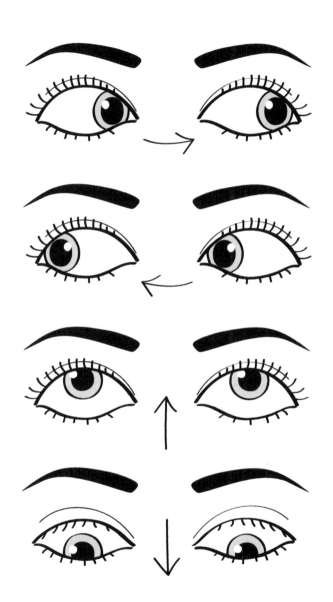

EXERCISE 9

Swinging

**Swing your eyes from side to side
four times, then up and down four times,
looking as far as you can in each direction.**

Do this as often as you can throughout the day.

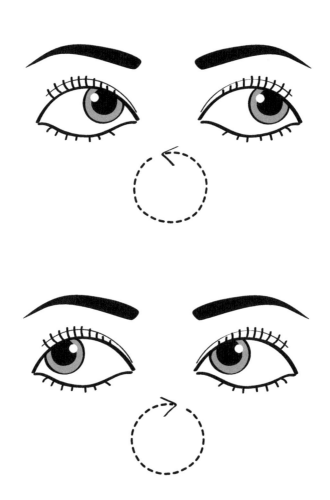

EXERCISE 10

Circles

**Swivel your eyes round and round
– four times in one direction, then four
times in the other, always striving to see
as far as possible in all directions.**

Do this as often as you can throughout the day.

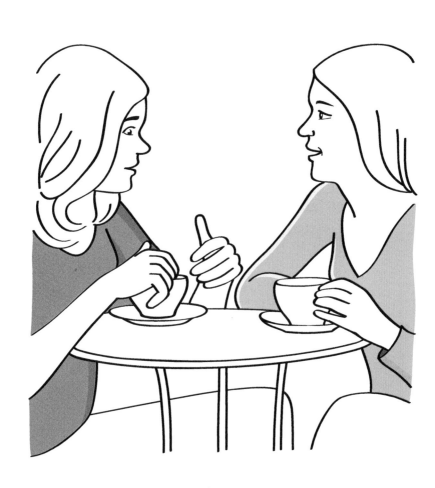

EXERCISE 11

Break the staring habit

Break the staring habit.
Keep your eyes moving in small shifts
all the time. Just don't stare.

Whenever you are looking at something or someone, keep your eyes moving in small shifts.

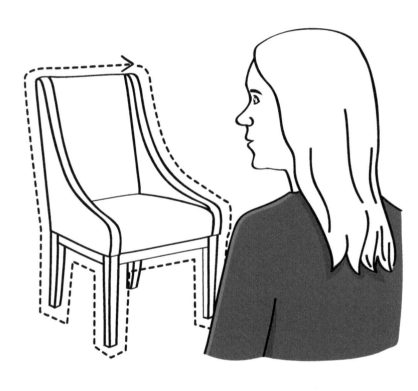

EXERCISE 12

Outlining

**With your eyes, follow the outline of
any object within clear view – perhaps
a table, a chair, or even a tree – first
clockwise and then anti-clockwise.**

Get into the habit of doing this as often as possible
throughout the day.

Lightning Source UK Ltd.
Milton Keynes UK
UKOW07f0505031116
286788UK00010B/25/P